POLIO

POST POLIO

SYNDROME

By

Anne Elizabeth Nixon

DEDICATION

To all those who love life,

see the bright side,

want to be free

and soar

above

pain,

I

dedicate

these pages

meant to help you.

Your friend, Anne Nixon

PREFACE

Seldom has a disease frightened an entire country like polio did when I was growing up in the 1930s and '40s. Our president, Franklin Delano Roosevelt, had polio as a young man, and was confined to a wheelchair, though without television, few people were aware of his painful and debilitated condition. Photographers shot waist-up pictures and never showed his hips or legs in a wheelchair.

You may be a survivor or the relative or friend of one. Be thankful if you lived after having this disease, for many haven't been so fortunate. Your story may be similar to mine, but in its own way different, too. You'll recognize many of the changes and feelings I've had over the years, and certainly by chance or design, have forgotten some.

It's strange how the mind pushes away things we need to forget. I learned of one such occurrence when my sister told me a story I'd archived into that Don't Remember part of my brain.

One day I told her how odd it was that I was afraid of looking at the wheels and pulleys at the top of elevators. In old buildings there are occasionally metal mesh cages for elevators, and I always hung onto someone's hand and kept my eyes down when near them or, heaven forbid, had to get into one.

"Well, you know why that is," she cried, astounded I'd say such a thing.

"No."

"You mean you don't remember when we were little and got stuck in that elevator between floors at the—"

"What?!!!!"

Nancy laughed, sure I was kidding her. But when I didn't answer she realized I really didn't know.

"I was too young to be able to do anything," she said, "but you were about eight maybe, and a man on the elevator opened the little door in the ceiling. He held you up so you could crawl on top and open the door to the next floor."

She looked at me and I looked at her.

"You're kidding!"

"No. I'm not."

She must have seen the horrified look on my face, and finally realized I'd placed that terrifying experience somewhere that I wouldn't have to confront it ever again. And if that conversation hadn't come up between us,

I never would have. I still can't look at all that horrendous equipment, but at least I know why.

That may be how you've felt about some of your polio experiences…

CHAPTER ONE

I watched my drive as it flew left, wishing the little golf ball could have gone to the right. That was where the cart path was. I could drive the cart along and simply get out, walk a few steps, hit my ball again and scoot back in again. But now I'd have to walk thirty or more painful, unsteady steps to the #$%^& ball nestled in the recently-mowed grass!

Only a year and a half before I was walking the course, pushing my bag of clubs, wishing for a good drive, but not aching for one. It had progressed from no balance problems to a slight one, but all of a sudden my problems had leaped like a jack rabbit.

On that sunny, and consequently happy outdoor sport day in the Northwest I hobbled out to my golf cart. I'd begun taking a simple pain pill before playing, which was pretty new to me. But it helped me get through two to three hours of more-than-usual activity once or twice a week.

At the end of the fifth hole where the cart path was fifty feet from the green, I had to speak up.

"This is it," I said to those nearest me. "I can't go on."

No one understood, of course, that I meant forever, never again would I be out there playing golf with them!

It all began many years before, my downhill slide. That's only apparent now, for at the time I had supposed it was the normal process of becoming older. But mine was different from my friends' aging, whether I knew it or not.

For ten years my husband, Don, and I motor-homed, "full-timers" the popular name had become. We hauled a canoe and two bicycles on top of our little Volkswagen tow car and I helped lift them onto the rack without trouble. When we parked our RV, we began exploring the surrounding area. As we walked miles every day, my legs never tired.

But the last year we were on the road I had trouble with my right hip, like it was out of joint. An x-ray showed my hip ball and socket were intact though. Only after we stopped our traveling in 1996 did I seek help with my discomfort. The doctor had me sit on the examining table and he swung my lower leg from side to side.

It's your hip joint," he said. "You'll need an x-ray, but I feel sure it will show you should have your hip replaced."

And that was the beginning of what I began recognizing as my decline.

In the hospital I asked the doctor, "May I see the hip joint you remove?" I'd worked in doctors' offices and also at Oregon's medical school, so I had seen a great many x-rays. But this one would be mine.

 "Certainly."

So one morning a tall, thin pathologist carrying a rectangular white metal pan stood at my hospital door. "I have your joint," he said, smiling.

He helped me understand what I saw by pointing out one completely flat side of the bone that should have been round (normally the round ball rotates in a round space or socket).

"You have no arthritis." Then pointing to the flat side, he remarked, "It's just worn away over here." I've wondered what he might have said if he'd known I'd had polio years before. But he didn't, and I had no idea I should have mentioned it.

After returning home from that operation a friend cautioned me, "You'd look better if you didn't lean forward from your waist. It's kind of old looking."

I thanked her and tried to stand up straighter. Good posture had always been something I'd taken for granted, and I didn't want to slump now that I had recently turned sixty!

Nothing changed for quite a few years after the surgery, and whether I continued leaning forward, I'm not sure. My friend moved away and no one mentioned it. I walked miles and dug and pulled up razor clams at the ocean beach, gardened for as many hours as I wanted, and golfed—all without discomfort. While others had aches and pains, joint replacements, and took pain medications, I had no more problems. In fact, I was the healthiest, and oldest, in my large family.

But then, little by little I found myself buying a small bottle of pain medication. When I hurt I reached for one of the soft ice packs I kept in the freezer, and leaned against it in that sore spot. Those two things kept me happy and what I considered "healthy."

Eventually I began making appointments with a chiropractor. At first they were a month or more apart, whenever my neck and back seemed to be "out." I told him about my polio, but still didn't recognize the progression of my disease, called post-polio syndrome. In fact, I'd never heard that term then.

From monthly appointments with the chiropractor I progressed over a few years to weekly ones. Every Monday at 10 o'clock I drove the ten miles down our narrow peninsula to his office, enjoyed his jokes and felt so much better as I left.

However, within the last year or two, every so often as I left I'd turn around and come back in.

"My back went out as I walked to the car," I'd complain.

So up I'd go again onto his table for another adjustment, hoping it would stay that time.

Just before he took early retirement, and prior to my giving up golf, several times I had to get back on the table for the doctor to redo my adjustment as soon as he'd finished—before leaving his office. It simply wouldn't stay.

Within the month of September of 2015, three things happened almost simultaneously. My wonderful, pain-saving chiropractor retired; I quit golfing; I gave my clubs to a granddaughter with the words, "I hope you'll enjoy these as much as I have." I knew that would keep me from giving in and getting out on that beautiful green course again—probably for a few short weeks, or days, or hours…

**

I'm going to tell you my story from the onset of symptoms to the "downhill slide" I just finished. But first, let me give you a little polio history:

Poliomyelitis, or infantile paralysis, was rampant in the late 1930s, 1940s, and 1950s, before vaccines. In the United States, as in the rest of the world, it struck the muscles of children and adults, rendering them useless or debilitated.

Eventually it was determined to be a virus, but without knowledge of prevention or cure, swimming pools and beaches closed, believing they might be the breeding grounds. Everything was in the "what if" and "maybe" stage.

Hot spring spas became popular centers when doctors discovered warm water and massage benefited patients who survived. They had been a favorite spot for the rich to relax and enjoy life, but turned into areas overrun with nurses and rehabilitation therapists.

In those days of great fear, we all knew someone who was struck down with polio, some who never returned to school, church or work again, and others who died within days. The most dreadful type I heard of as a young person was what attacked the lungs. We understood it struck with swiftness and if the patient survived long enough to get to an iron lung, it was miraculous.

A young high school boy who lived in Chicago overlooking Lake Michigan swam almost daily in the lake which was so large it appeared more like a bay or ocean. On Thursday afternoon he changed into his bathing suit and dove in for a quick swim before beginning his homework.

By Sunday he was dead.

Polio attacked his lungs and in the hospital his fever rose and rose. His parents were very wealthy, but money could do nothing. And he was a big, healthy young man—again that was immaterial. The viral disease consumed him. So he was never helped by an iron lung, which is a ventilator that enables a patient to breathe when his normal muscle is destroyed. He didn't live long enough for that.

One survivor was a little girl in my grade school at the beginning of the outbreak. I was about ten. When she was absent our teacher told us of her serious disease. About a year later she returned with a huge metal brace on her stricken leg. It clicked at her knee as she walked very slowly. Jane was a small girl, and it must have been a heavy burden, both literally and figuratively.

Nowadays polio originating in our country is unheard of. The first preventive step was the Sabin vaccine which was a liquid and dropped onto sugar cubes. Then came the stronger vaccinations by Salk which most of us remember. That pretty well rid us of polio since the late 1970s.

This first photo below is one like polio patients were placed into in the 1940s and 50s, very different from the second picture that looks modern in comparison.

I'm amazed this little girl is smiling, for it seems like being constricted and unable to run around and play would be very, very sad—and mighty difficult.

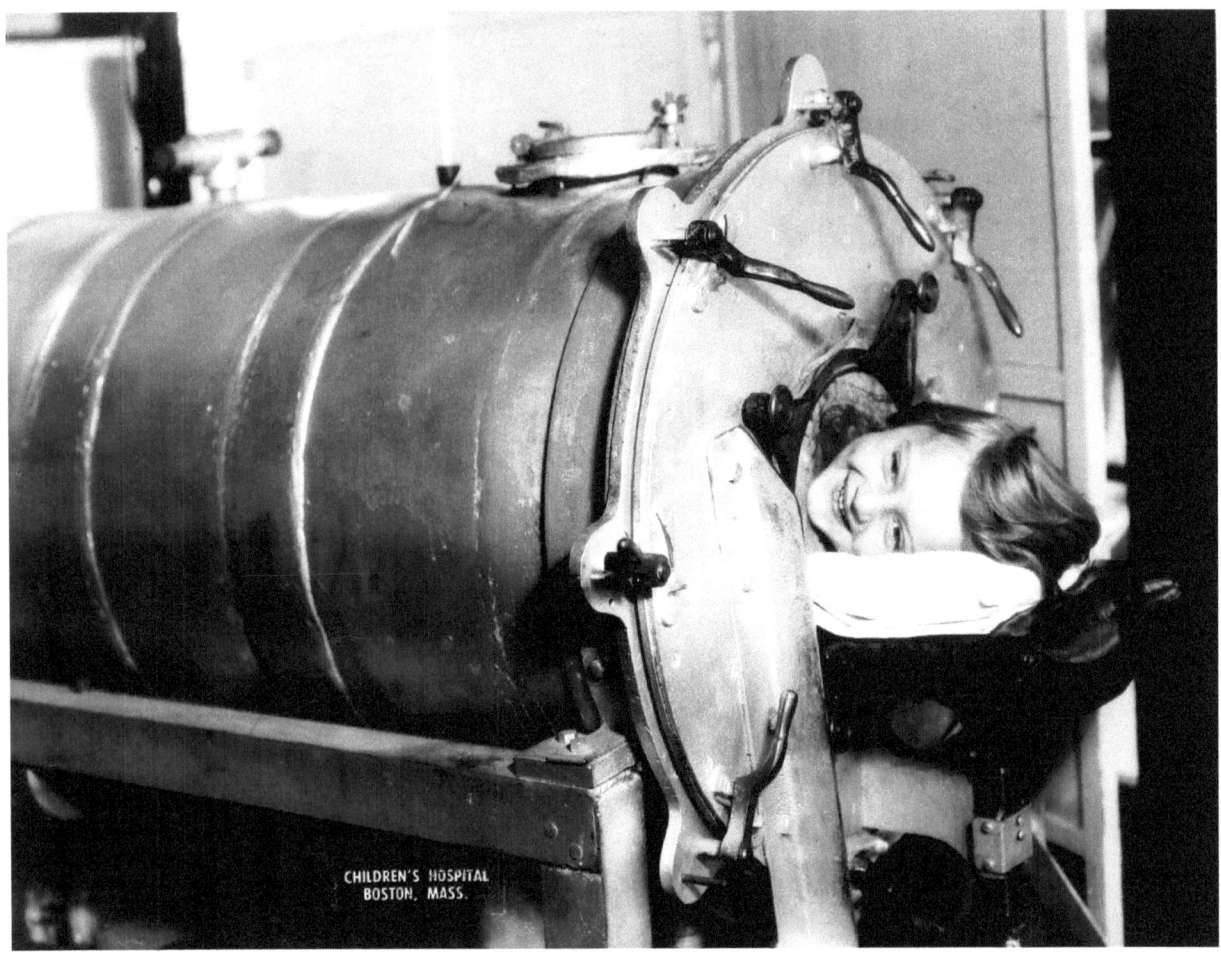

CHILDREN'S HOSPITAL
BOSTON, MASS.

The only person I've known who survived an iron lung is a writer friend and she described to me the feeling of being confined. She lived that way for over one year. When I knew her she was middle-aged and limped quite visibly as she used a cane—possibly in constant pain. I never felt it polite to ask her all the questions I might have, but now wish I had.

Recently I've been surprised to learn of two people who are in their sixties and had polio. They live active lives, and probably that's why they amaze me, for I'd never have suspected. They didn't have any left-over symptoms like my writer friend. In fact, one has the throwing arm of an outfielder, a woman! But then I think about the fact that no one would have suspected I'd had polio either.

Where I now live I've come to know a woman who has seen symptoms much the same as mine. Each of us were misdiagnosed at the time of our illness too.

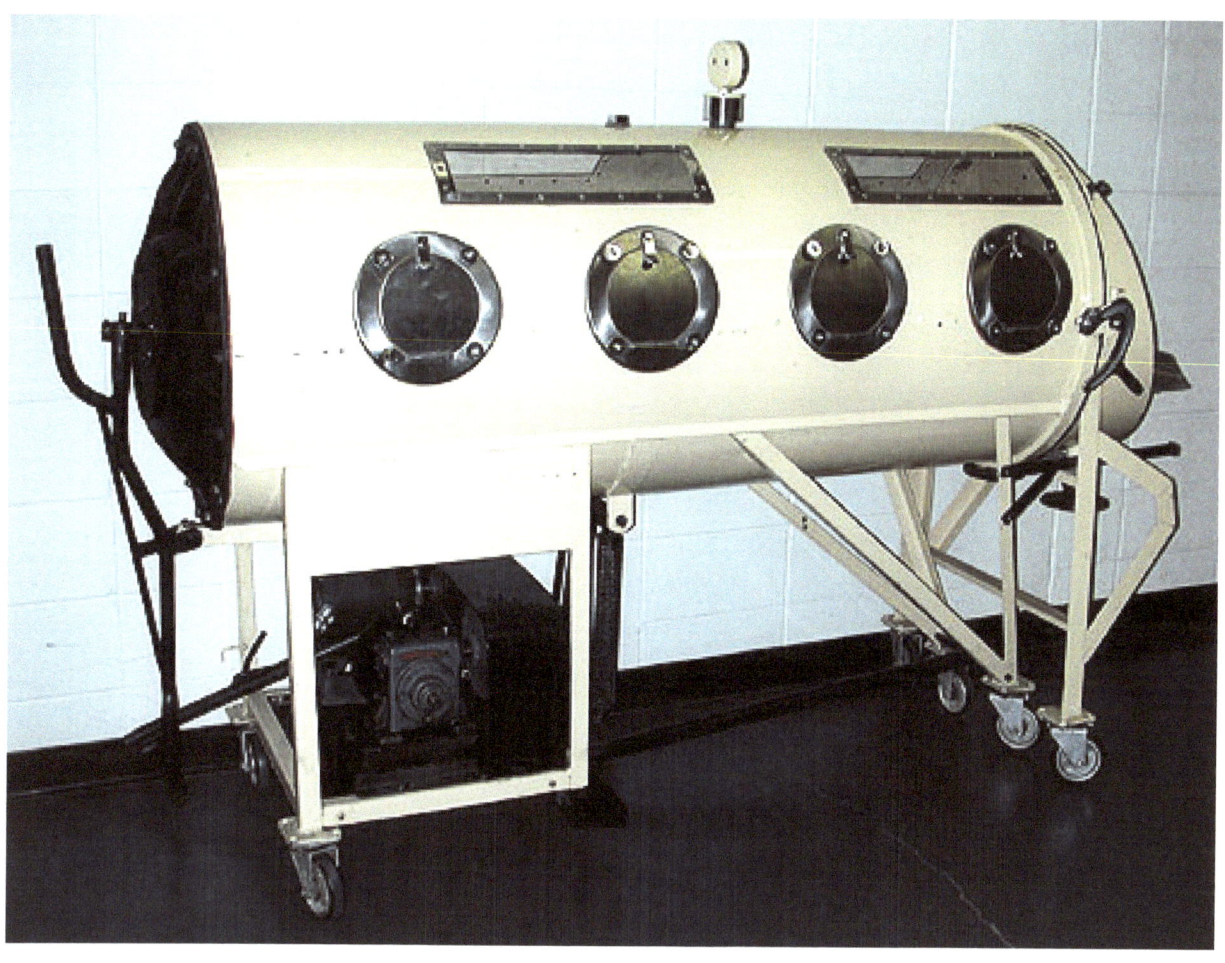

This iron lung looks a lot more modern than the other which resembles an old barrel.

CHAPTER TWO

When I was twenty, married and with a baby almost a year old, I contracted polio. The days before I was hospitalized were eerie. As I look back, it was more like fiction than fact.

In 1954 drive-in movies were popular, and in Colorado Springs, CO I sat in a car with my husband and baby, Davy. At intermission my husband walked to the "bar" for coffee, and handed me a cup when he returned. I sat in the front seat with the coffee in my right hand, until suddenly the hot liquid had spilled all over me. There was no bumping my hand or wrist, nothing. My hand simply gave way—and fortunately Davy was asleep in the back seat and not on my lap.

By the next day I felt seriously ill, but not debilitated. It was different from any illness, for I wasn't nauseated, did not hurt, could get up without discomfort. But I knew I was ill.

My husband was in the Army Signal Corps, stationed at Fort Carson. I said to myself, I must get his fatigues and dress uniforms ironed, for I know I won't have time to do that in the future. I'll be in the hospital. It was not a dramatic statement, just a truthful one. I knew instinctively that I would not be home. So I got the uniforms ready, then spent the afternoon ironing, readying myself for what was to come.

(In those days sprinkling bottles were standard for ironing. Mine was an empty catsup bottle with a stopper full of tiny holes I'd bought and stuck into the top. Filling the bottle with water, I tipped it and wet down the clothes, then rolled them up in a towel and gave them an hour to "meld" moisture.) I set up my ironing board, heated my iron—no steam irons in those days—to cotton, and began my job.

After a couple of hours I got dinner ready, fed Davy, and went to bed, exhausted.

"I want you to take me to the hospital," I told my husband the next morning.
"You sick?" he asked.
"Yes."
"What's the matter?"
"I'm sick," I repeated. There were no words to describe it.
So at the Army hospital I saw a young doctor who told me, "We'll get blood tests and x-rays, but I believe you have spinal meningitis."
That sounded ominous, and I asked, "What's that?"

"Inflammation of the spinal column and brain," he told me, avoiding much explanation.

"Will it make me go crazy?"

"Oh, no." (I've often hoped that made an impression on him and he gave longer answers from then on!)

A nurse eased me into a wheelchair, and we took off through barren, gray halls. But they were busy in the x-ray department and I remember sitting slumped in the big, wooden wheelchair for what seemed like many, many hours as I waited, though I'm sure it wasn't hours long. After that was over I was introduced to another aide who pushed me to a surgical unit for a spinal tap. No one thought of keeping me segregated at any stage.

When my tests were over a nurse wheeled me into a huge empty room of beds with white sheets and pillows. As she helped me get out of the wheel chair and down between cool sheets, the relief of lying flat was lovely, something I remember to this day.

But I was there in error and soon went to isolation. It was a private room, and whenever a person came in they put on a clean gown and mask. I stayed there for two weeks, and I recall nothing but severe headaches and pain all over. What I ate, whether I went for more tests or had them administered in my room, I have no idea.

The only thing I do know is that my husband and baby were given gamma globulin shots, hopefully to prevent them from catching my illness. Davy was banned from coming to see me, and was cared for by our neighbor landlady who had three children of her own.

But I had no worries, for I slept those days away, unaware of anything.

However, eventually I looked out the window that lay only a few feet from my bed. As I became more aware, to leave the hospital became a goal and I spent hours plotting my escape. Maybe I could slide a chair over, open the window and climb out. Lack of energy kept me bedbound, though. How long would I have to stay? I never asked. Lethargy overtook me.

At the end of those two weeks, just before Davy's first birthday in November, I did return home to our tiny two room converted trailer. But I was far from well. My body was stiff and weak. An oil heater helped me warm my legs which tightened and cramped often, making it impossible to sit, for my muscles were too tight to bend for more than a few minutes. Sleeping was difficult, too. So off and on, day and night, I returned to the warmth of our stove to sooth my muscles. A month later my husband was discharged and we returned to Oregon.

My parents saw my thin, weak body and urged us to stay with them rather than look for a house. They also asked if I'd go to their physician who had made a study of poliomyelitis. (Remember, I had been diagnosed with spinal meningitis.)

"I believe you had polio, not meningitis," the doctor told me. "Your muscles need strengthening."

That meant going to a rehabilitation center three times a week for an hour, twelve hours of sleep each night, a nap every afternoon, and no baby lifting for six months. No driving—someone would have to take me to the Rehab Center for massage and lifting weights.

At rehabilitation I heard, "Have someone suspend ropes through pulleys with weights, maybe in your basement." So my father and husband set up my weight-lifting equipment downstairs for me. But I used it only sporadically for my lethargy left me uncaring and ineffective. I recovered in spite of myself!

My mother, who was going back to school to renew her teaching certificate after many years, took over caring for Davy, never complaining. I remember little of it all, perhaps by design. But I did get well and stronger.

"It's important you always keep active. If you slack off, it will be your great loss," Dr. Wilson told me, adding ominously, **"then your strength might never return."** I was lucky and thankful. I'd always been active and vowed to be forever. I'm thankful I at least listened to that, for I was not what you'd call athletic.

CHAPTER THREE

With a pain-free life I seldom needed painkillers. Many of you will have conditions that necessitate different drugs, but I've been very fortunate, and until after middle-age, only occasional meds have been required. I remember having a severe case of strep throat, my first and only, but responded well to antibiotic therapy just as I would have if I'd never had polio.

Another bit of luck is having been born with a positive attitude. I don't wake up wondering how I'll look at life. One day for me is like all the rest: wonderful!

If you have trouble keeping your spirits up it's important to seek help. It will make your post-polio syndrome much easier to accept and tolerate. Talk to your doctor about it and see what he suggests. Follow his directions or find another doctor who understands how post-polio affects those of us who are having more problems, or different ones, than some of his other patients.

Keep as active as you possibly can. We have many gyms nowadays with a variety of exercise equipment. If that's too expensive, an exercise bicycle, new or used from a secondhand shop, can be set up in your home. If you're able to ride a regular bike, that gets you out in the fresh air as well as using your muscles. Whatever you do, though, move!

Not all of us are able to use exercise equipment. If you are able to use your legs at all, look for a **small pedal exerciser.** It sits on the floor in front and below a chair.

Keep in contact with your friends, old and new. That's fun and healthy for mind and spirit. It may be possible only by phone or internet, but make time several days a week to keep in touch with others. You might pick ones who are lonesome, alone, ill, or have a tendency toward depression. Brighten up their days. You'd be giving and receiving help.

Try your best to keep your weight to a healthy-for-you level. There are lots of foods that don't put on weight, like celery, broccoli, cucumber, watermelon, eggs, tomatoes, spinach, and many others. Get out your computer and Google to find ones that appeal to you. **Eating healthy foods** is important without adding empty calories that increase your weight. If you're unable to work off those calories it's especially important to be careful. Excess weight can cause us to "eat away" at our independence.

Is there something you love to eat? If so, incorporate it into your meals occasionally, or if it's cheap and healthy, gobble it down daily! I've always loved breakfast, and spent extra time chopping up veggies and apples to mix into scrambled eggs. I made enough coffee or tea to drink as much as I enjoy. What a way to start the day, I told myself happily! I was fortunate to have a husband who ate anything I set before him, but if you have to make two different menus, do it occasionally to spoil yourself, and it can be any meal, not just breakfast. Maybe he can learn to cook and spoil you—are those your outrageous laughs ?!

Getting enough sleep makes everyone feel better, but it's very important for us with post-polio syndrome. If you can't go to bed earlier or get up later, try a nap at some point during the day. I'm not a napper, but also not a night owl, so I get enough sleep by turning in early. I need more sleep than many who are older than I. And often I get in bed to watch TV or read because I'm tired and it feels so good to lie down.

Rather than dwelling on illness or progression of your condition, **keep your mind on things you can change or enjoy, on others, or on projects you might have going.**

Don't be afraid to ask for help when necessary. That's hard for some of us to do. However, think of how much pleasure you get from helping others when you are able. They will feel that way in response to your needs.

Independence—try to keep it if you have it, or at least prolong the time you will lose it. There are things that we want to avoid, and falling is probably top on that list! As we age, any fall can qualify as a disaster, but with post-polio syndrome our muscles may not be strong enough to bounce back like others. So as you read this book, think about how a cane or walker can keep you on your feet.

Lastly, **keep a book (or your Kindle) ready for free moments**. That will encourage you to take a break because you'll WANT to sit down long enough to read a few pages. (I got myself a refurbished Kindle after ordering what I thought was a regular book. Then I discovered it was an e-book! So I bought what I needed to read it, and have been using it ever since. What did I do before I had it, I ask myself!) But

I must warn you, don't let yourself spend the day in a chair. **Give yourself a quick break, then get on with your day. <u>Inactivity could be your worst enemy!</u>**

CHAPTER FOUR

In the years after I recovered I don't remember thinking about my illness. Life was busy. My husband went back to school and I worked to support us. Davy was an easy boy to raise, interested in sports as he grew tall and later he loved cars. When he was in junior high, which meant about 15 years after my polio, I rose early enough to walk to his school's track with our dog so I could jog on a proper surface. For about half an hour I ran around, not fast, but at a speed that felt comfortable. That exercise was exhilarating, good for my psyche and offset my sedentary half-day job. When I see joggers zipping along a concrete sidewalk I cringe, for that's hard on joints. If you are able to walk, swing those arms and keep your eyes aimed ahead of you! And think about what you're seeing, like flowers, tall trees, cows in a field, the color of cars on a busy street—whatever makes your walk interesting. Maybe you have a dog that would like to go for a daily stroll, too.

In 1978, over thirty years after my polio, I easily hiked ten miles into a week-long camping trip. Part of it was steep, but most on a level plane. We carried our personal belongings on our backs but the rest was hauled in by pack horses, making it easier on us all.

Then six years later Don and I joined the same group for another week of camping. That was completely different terrain, and we gazed across deep ravines at mountain goats, which is how we felt ourselves!

To initially get to our campsite we began with a steep climb, so coming down it was just as tough on our muscles and joints. During the week we went on daily hikes, which is where we spied the goats. This was extreme and I don't expect many of you to do such a thing. My father was a mountain climber and it was a group of hikers I'd grown up knowing. Otherwise, I'm sure I wouldn't have even begun to consider such a hike. I doubt any of them were aware I'd had polio, and at that time I felt as though I never had had that disease.

(A little aside: On one of our long day hikes where a drop-off to our left felt scary, the woman in front of Don tripped. He grabbed for her and pulled her back onto the trail!)

That was the last hike like that I ever took, but I mention it to encourage those of you who are able, to push yourselves. If you live in an area that's hilly it could be possible; but many don't, and those exercise machines are a good alternative.

In 1995, the winter before we quit RVing, we house-sat for my sister and her husband. It became the perfect time to buy used furniture with many "twisty" chair legs and parts to refinish for the house we intended to buy. That meant a great deal of sanding, and being right-handed, I used my right hand, the side of my polio weakening. Several years later the joints of that hand began thickening and twisting; while not achy, I appeared to have severe arthritis. A doctor who I never thought to tell about my polio history, assured me it was only stress arthritis, but I now believe it may have been the first of my post-polio problems, like my hip that was discovered a year later. Those fingers have never been painful like osteoarthritis, but anyone seeing my fingers would expect I had a lot of discomfort.

When you have some new condition, if there's any possibility it could be affecting you because of your post-polio, mention that to your doctor or whoever you're consulting.

My belief is that life should be lived in whatever way gives us happiness. For example, my son, called Dave instead of Davy as he grew older, bought a motorcycle after he was 18 and decided to take a trip with a good friend. They left Oregon and headed south on the Pacific Coast Highway into California, then east to Nevada and north again. A friend asked me, "Don't you worry yourself to death having to think about such a trip?"

I've always taken for granted my upbeat attitude toward life. "As long as he's doing what makes him happy, I believe that's important," I told her.

Being overcautious, wishing he or she could do something but being afraid, robs us of much of the joy we could get from life. The same is true of how we treat our post-polio symptoms. Try to do as much as you can. There are many people with far more debilitating problems and at all ages. So try not to dwell on the changes in your life, but do as much as you're able.

Could our post-polio syndrome be affected by being unhappy with life? Possibly. Don't give that a chance! Enjoy every day!

There are a few things I've changed during the past six or eight years. One is knitting and hand sewing because it produced pain. I gave all my knitting supplies away, and though I missed it, other things took its place. With sewing, I found a bright and cheery compact sewing box where I keep only what I need for replacing buttons and basic necessities. I seldom have to use it, but when I do I make it as simple and quick as I can.

Recently I used a needle and thread for about 15 minutes and had a good deal of discomfort because I used my "bad" hand. (If it had been something I could have performed with the other hand, I'd have done that as I do with many projects.) After a few hours, however, it was gone because I used a roll-on pain reliever. If it hadn't been taken care of that way, I'd have smeared some more on over the knuckles that hurt. I have added the roll-on recently after realizing how quick and easy it is. When I find something I know I'll use, rather than putting it off and enduring pain unnecessarily, I buy it if it's a sensible price.

Another is the shoes I wear. Good support and comfort mean a lot to people like us. And interested, competent clerks who check our joints and toes to be sure they are where they belong for a good fit are invaluable. I pay more now, but they are quality shoes with sufficient arch support and I keep them for many years. If you have lifts be very sure you are conscientious about using them. In the last few years I have had to change my shoes due to neuropathy; I have pain if my toes are covered. You may discover different reasons for special shoes, but be sure they are comfortable on your feet. Remember, you are fortunate to be able to walk, and your feet are what propel you!

You may begin using a cane. Buy a sturdy one. Some have curved tops and others a 90-degree-angle. Others have three prongs on the bottom for support, and some can stand by themselves when you need your hands for something for a few moments. With no idea what length a cane should be, ask your doctor or therapist. My daughter-in-law wondered why I held onto it on the opposite side of my weakness, and I told her, "I have no idea. I'll ask the doctor about it when I go in." So I did, and he said I was correct. Evidently we hold it whichever side helps us most. As you keep your shoulders back, be careful not to raise them for that's unnatural. If you are using a walker, the same is true. Whatever you use, try to stand as straight (and healthy) as you can.

I've vowed not to leave the house without some form of help, such as a cane. It's easy to tell yourself it's okay just this once for snipping a bouquet or clipping off a dead blossom.

There should never be an exception.

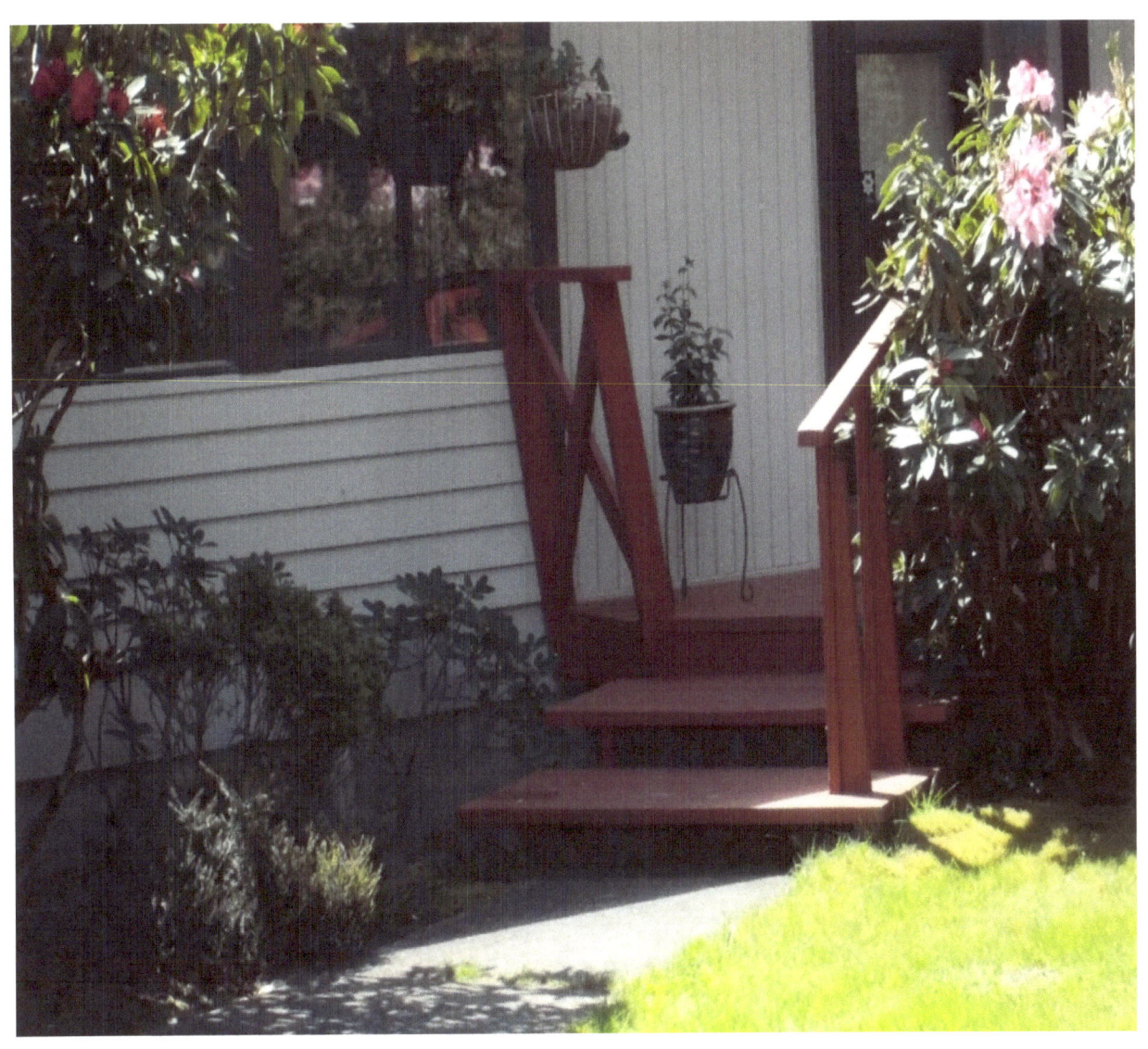

LONG, DEEP STEPS ARE EASIER FOR CANES & WALKERS.

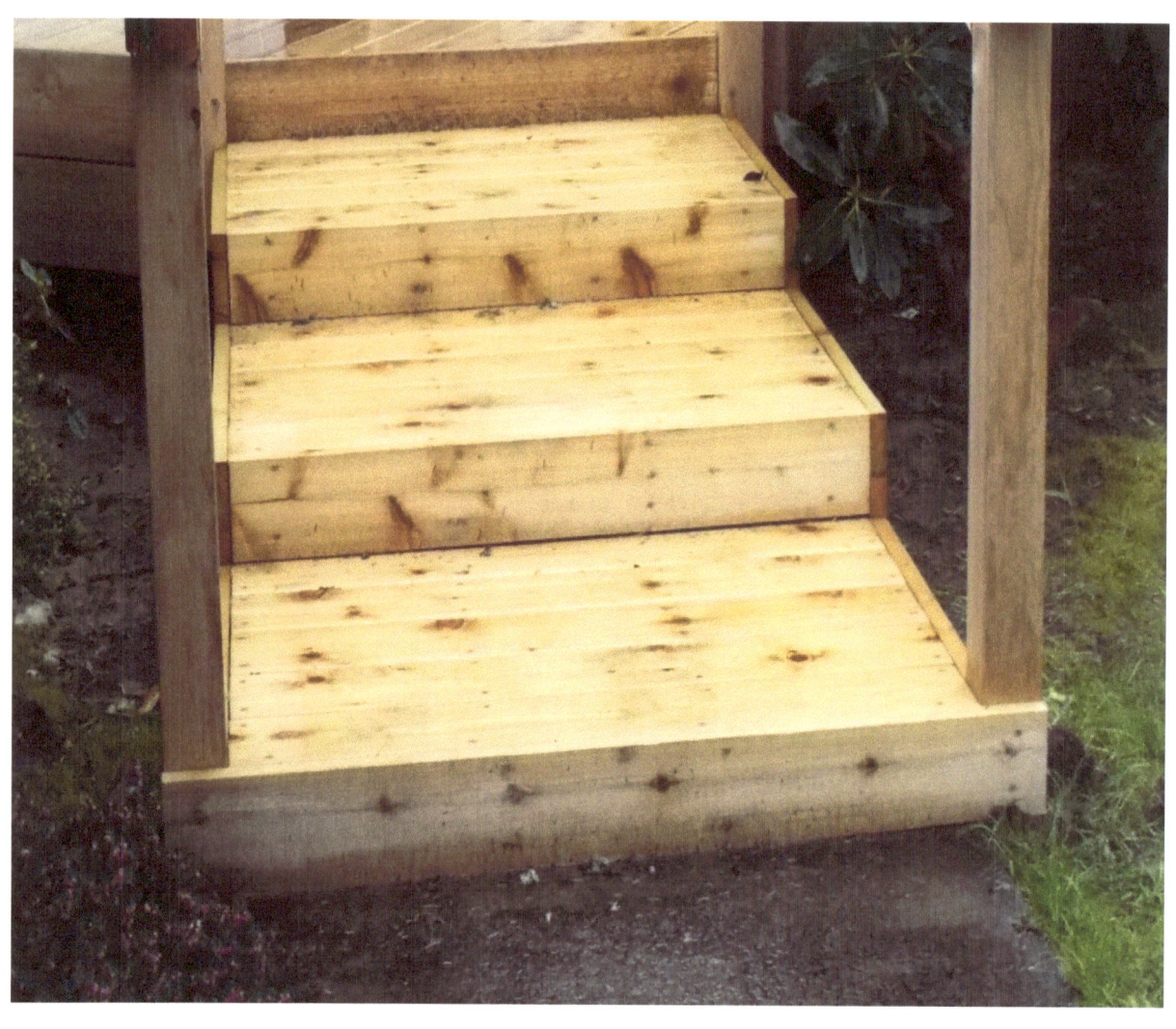

THE FRONT STEPS WERE REBUILT AND WE ADDED A HAND RAIL ON THE LEFT AS WELL AS THE ORIGINAL ONE ON THE RIGHT SIDE.

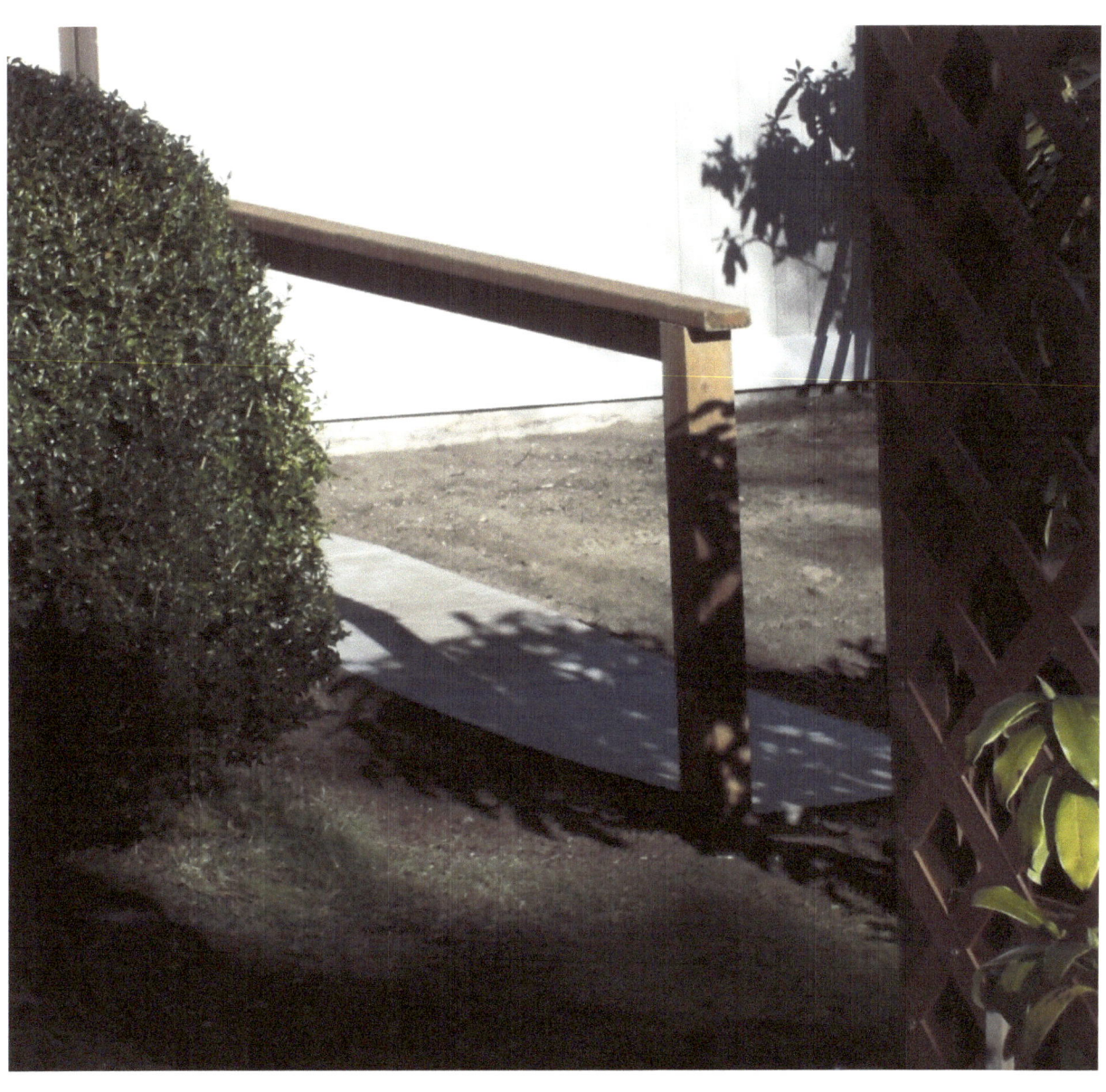

FOR UNEVEN, SLOPING GROUND, CEMENT SQUARES AND HANDRAILS MAKE A SAFER WAY TO ENJOY THE OUTDOORS.

ODDS AND ENDS:

Within the last year my right wrist has gone the way of the rest of my body. There are few ways I can use my right hand now without discomfort, and I've found I can be ambidextrous. I eat with my left hand, and use my knife with my right hand to push food onto the fork, keeping my wrist straight.

Due to pain during the night in my right wrist I decided to invest in a 2-inch band for compression and to keep it in line while I'm asleep. It helps a great deal.

With a big, long-handled ladle I bought online, I scoop out new, clean cat litter from an open cloth bag, after having help dumping it into that bag from the plastic one it came in. For a while I cleaned up a lot of messes, but have become pretty adept at the job.

Writing is painful and eventually I may have to write with my left hand. I will change my signature with the bank when I can't sign my name. **Be sure to notify those who will require your legal signature of a change and give them a sample of the "new you."**

A printer allows me to be my old-fashioned self and write letters when I want to, especially important for friends who don't have computers for online correspondence. Those letters can be as long as I want, too. When and if I discover it's too painful to use my right hand for typing I'll look into a computer I can speak into, for that's now a possibility.

When I had my right hip replaced I asked the orthopedist if he could be sure **both legs would be the same length** because I knew there was a slight difference. He told me he could if it were little enough, which it was. But if the leg on your polio-affected side is several inches shorter, I understand they can elongate it now. Be sure to look into it. If not, you can have one shoe changed into a wedge-type. Or if you buy a wedge shoe, one could be made higher than the other. Don't be afraid people will see it, for I'll bet no one cares, or maybe they'll admire you for what you are able to do.

A doctor warned me many years ago, "**Never have a spinal anesthesia,**" unless absolutely necessary. For one surgery I learned that was what the surgeon preferred but I refused it and asked that the information be put on the front of my chart. Nowadays charts aren't paper, but the warning can still be included in your important Allergy section.

CHAPTER FIVE

We survivors should be proud of our status, and in another decade will hopefully be a rare breed in the U.S. But Africa is still finding new cases. When I first began losing my balance I suspected it might be from polio. I called for an appointment at the University of Oregon's medical school, OHSU, and was seen in the Neurology Department. The doctor who examined me was an outstanding man. Unfortunately, he has passed away, but each year during his vacation he traveled to Africa to treat and study polio victims. At that appointment he confirmed my suspicion, and told me I did have post-polio syndrome. He warned me about falling, but urged that I live life to the fullest.

To assure yourself you have adequate support for preventing tumbles, here are three suggestions:
Canes. This will probably be your first attempt.
Walkers. There are a great variety of styles, weights and sizes.
Rollators. These are similar to walkers but built heavier.

If you have trouble getting out of your easy chair, there are some that boost a person to an upright position, making it easy to get onto your feet. They are available at most furniture stores and online. This may be something to consider now or in the years to come. People of all ages find these helpful, but you must be careful not to fall forward as you stand and leave the chair.

Some of us eventually become wheelchair-bound, taking on symptoms of our disease again after many years. Many wheelchairs are light weight, which may be easier to get around in, as well as for transporting in the back seat or trunk of a car. The one pictured below, light weight, obviously needs someone to push it, or the person be able to move himself around with his feet. The ones frequently seen are heavier and most often pushed by someone walking behind, but can be used by a person with strong arms to push on the top of the wheels—allowing them to be independently mobile. There are others that have head and lower leg support, but otherwise serve the same purpose.

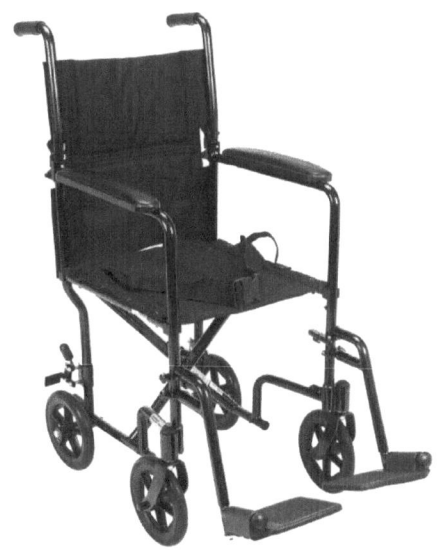

While you may not have had such a dramatic spiral downward, most of us continue losing ground. I now live in an assisted care facility after tearing my right medial meniscus (the innermost cartilage between the bones of my knee). My husband had Alzheimer's disease and until that tear I was able to help him enough to stay in our home. But, as you may also have discovered, sometimes circumstances bring life into CAPITAL LETTERS. It had been obvious we couldn't go on much longer the way we had been; my husband's disease had progressed significantly and my balance and getting-around problems had also.

When that injury struck I was off my feet, so with help we temporarily went to a nearby assisted care home, then moved to be near our children. My husband had come to the point of needing a memory care facility, and I was able to find one in the city where we planned to move.

{For your information: After the meniscus tear, I learned the following: there are injections of a gaseous nature which may relieve pain. They are given very specifically: one week apart three times. I say "may" because there's no way to tell until after at least the second week's injection if it is going to be successful. I opted to try, and found no difference after the second or third one. If it had worked I could have had another set of three shots after six months. Arthritis pain can be treated with this substance, too, I understand, administered by orthopedists. We are all subject to arthritis, no matter what our family history may be.}

I decided to see my doctor about neuropathy of my feet. At the time I had no idea it might increase to become a debilitating problem. It can be caused by diabetes, or as with mine, chemotherapy and radiation. As I lay on the couch recuperating from the chemo before surgery I often asked my husband to rub my feet because they tingled and hurt. Over the years it increased to the point I had trouble going to sleep. Since we with post-polio syndrome often have trouble walking we must be aware of this condition. My doctor told me the generic of Lyrica, gabapentin, might help. Upon taking a low dosage I've had relief and especially in the evening. This may or may not help you, but ask your doctor if you have neuropathy. And a caution: it may make you sleepy, so don't take it and drive or use machinery or anything that could hurt you.

In my assisted care facility I now use a walker, though previously, when going out I took my cane if I felt I'd be safe enough. Post-polio syndrome has progressed in my life, and it is something expected. I am always realistic about those changes. It may have begun when I came to grips with the fact I'd never be able to do what I used to, like climbing up on a riding lawn mower, or scooting in behind the wheel of a car. In fact, just walking out into our rural yard began to feel risky. It's not easy for a person who is independent. But I know I've been extremely fortunate and we all must realize there are so many people in worse condition than we are. Tiny changes occur that we may not notice until they increase. Life is often a balancing act. Don't forget what you're thankful for. If you get discouraged, as we all do occasionally, make a mental or virtual list of the Good Things. Positive thoughts are healing. They stimulate endorphins in our bodies which are a healing force.

Two years have passed since I wrote this book, and life has changed dramatically in some ways, but little in others. I should get more sleep and rest than I did even one year ago, but I often don't get it until I try to read and drop off to doze for a little while. I've been taking Melatonin that I find helps me sleep, a hormone from the pineal gland in the brain. So if you have trouble with your sleep, you might ask your doctor about it. But also beware, it is not sleep apnea that is completely different and not in any way related.

I live with close to 100 people, many who are older than I, and a few who need a lot of care by aides. There are a few who simply prefer to stay in their apartments all day and have meals delivered by the kitchen, though medically they could come out to eat. I have preferences, so some days I'm quite active and others less so. But I try to do as my body dictates, occasionally going to bed by 8 PM to watch TV. It feels so very good to lie down! And I have a lovely little kitty I enjoy spending time with.

My husband passed away in the spring of 2018, and while I miss him so very much, I know it is a blessing that he isn't suffering any more.

Since my husband's death I decided it was time to look into the repair of my right knee, the one in which I tore the meniscus. The orthopedist had x-rays taken, then told me what I could have done for the pain—cortisone injections or replacement.

"I have no pain," I told him. "I use this walker or a cane because I lack balance, and I thought that was due to the meniscus tear."

The orthopedist explained the three x-rays showed evidence of arthritis, a great surprise, for I've always been happy to have been one without painful arthritis.

He explained the problem I have getting around is no doubt due to my post-polio disease. I'd supposed the meniscus tear had been the cause of my need for a walker, because it was after that injury that I began using it.

So even if I'd had the meniscus tear repaired just after it happened, I'd still be needing the walker for the underlying polio disease.

I can almost hear your voices! "That's just like me!"

The other day our activity/exercise gal was asking questions. One was, "What are you thankful for?" My answer was, "That I don't need a wheelchair." Another lady in the class who had also had polio, said, "Amen!" To you, I'll say, **be thankful for all you DON'T have!** When the time comes, if it does, you'll be happy to have the wheelchair, but until then, use those legs as often as possible! And if you use a walker, try to stand up as straight as you can, not bending over. Placing your feet under the walker as far as is comfortable allows you to stand straighter. And if your back aches after walking or exercise, there are roll-on analgesics to roll onto the sore areas. I use them and feel so much better that I can participate in things I couldn't otherwise.

Since the time above, several things have begun happening. I'll add them here:

My right wrist began aching, a continuous ache that I sometimes notice, and other times not, depending upon what I'm doing. But at night in bed I try to lie with it in a position that won't hurt (naturally). What I mean by that is so that it won't wake me later if it begins to be more painful. I find letters missing in my typing, and usually they are those of my right hand (the post-polio side). My neck will turn only so far to the right without pain.

I have just ordered a knee brace with copper implanted into the material for my right knee. Over the past month or so I've noticed times when that knee pops or hurts as I walk. Occasionally without walking, just changing from bent to straight will cause that. I'm going to wear this every day as a precaution, <u>for I do everything I can to keep from getting worse due to my own negligence.</u> I urge you to do the same!

I'm adding this after almost a year from my last notes: I've been having more painful places as you no doubt are too. My right wrist and up into the outer area of my hand is almost always a painful problem, so I've gotten a copper wrist band and wear that quite often. It helps to some extent, but not entirely.

My left knee began having a painful spot on the outer side. It keeps me from standing up and sitting down, but doesn't hurt at all when still. Just what that is, I will hopefully find out when I see my doctor later this month. I tell you this so you will try to do something helpful about whatever it is that is bothering you. We all have different areas of discomfort and instead of just letting them hurt us, we should ask a doctor about the reasons.

A financial solution for post-polio syndrome folks might be this: Apply for a Reverse Mortgage to free up money to pay for assisted care, if you qualify. And long-term care insurance, which has to be done early, but it might be worth looking into. Be careful about the little details, however. I've heard of one that lasts only a <u>specified number of years</u>.

The most important thing I learned, as mentioned previously, is the statement the doctor told me so many years ago: "Always keep active. If you slack off, it will be your great loss. Then your strength might never return." Recently I mentioned this to the orthopedist—he agreed wholeheartedly.

I wish you all my very, very best! Enjoy your life, laugh a lot, be good to yourself and others, and be glad to be as healthy as you are!
Anne